This book Belongs to:

____

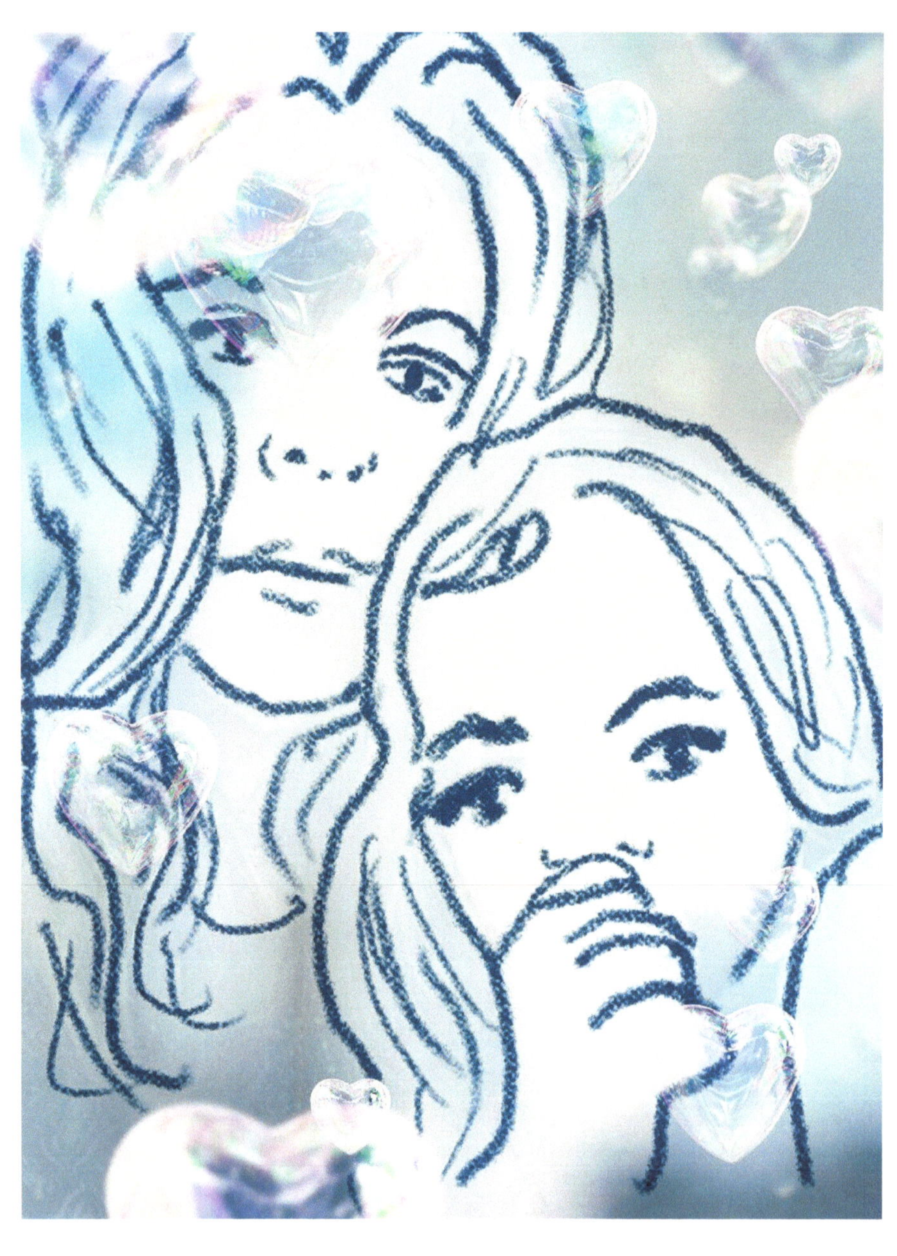

Hello I'm Sammy Grammy. I am a retired teacher.

I recently gained weight after retirement. It may be because during work I used to walk most of the day. I'm not quite as active now.

I had gained approximately 20 lbs. I really needed to lose 20 lbs. before I had gained the weight. So altogether I really needed to lose 40 lbs. to be in the middle of my BMI. BMI is body mass index. It's not the perfect way to evaluate weight but it helps.

Even when I was working I couldn't lose weight. I tried many diets.

I tried at least 10 diets. Sometimes I lost about 10 lbs. I struggled exercised etc. but I gained it back.

In 40 years I never really lost the weight and kept it off. I had steadily gained each year until I really was 40 lbs. overweight.

Does this sound familiar? Recently I had tried the low carb diet. I didn't lose weight and I didn't feel it was right for me. My sugar wasn't high and I'm watching my cholesterol and blood pressure. My blood pressure goal is to be under 120/85 and my cholesterol under 180. My doctor advised measuring my blood pressure 3 times a day for 3 weeks and keeping the results. Mine can vary 30 points in one day both diastolic and systolic. I'm aiming for under 120/85. I dont want to take medicine which is very expensive. I'm on a fixed income. I want to be healthy too.

My daughter was having problems with sugar. She tried the Keto diet. She lost a lot of weight but was sick a lot.

My daughter and I decided to try a vegan diet. With busy people that is really difficult. Vegan cooking takes a lot of work to make it eatable and sustainable.

Well to make things easy we started doing smoothies which were vegan. At first my daughter did vegan and I didn't stick with it very well.

My daughter was vegan for about 2 months when she began to feel better.

My daughter wasn't doing the diet to lose weight. She had already lost 30 lbs. She was doing this for autoimmune. Many ailments including diabetes, arthritis etc. are autoimmune. Some new studies seem to indicate autoimmune diseases are related and stem from an Epstein Barr virus.

https://www.healthline.com/health-news/how-mono-virus-can-raise-risk-of-lupus-and-other-autoimmune-diseases

I had begun doing smoothies in the AM everyday. I didn't lose any weight for about a month. My smoothie recipe is here. If you have any allergies you can change things. Make it vegan.

Sammy Grammy
Smoothie Recipe

Cashew milk
Celery or Kale
Frozen fruit (berries are
lowest carb)
any low carb fruit fresh
Water

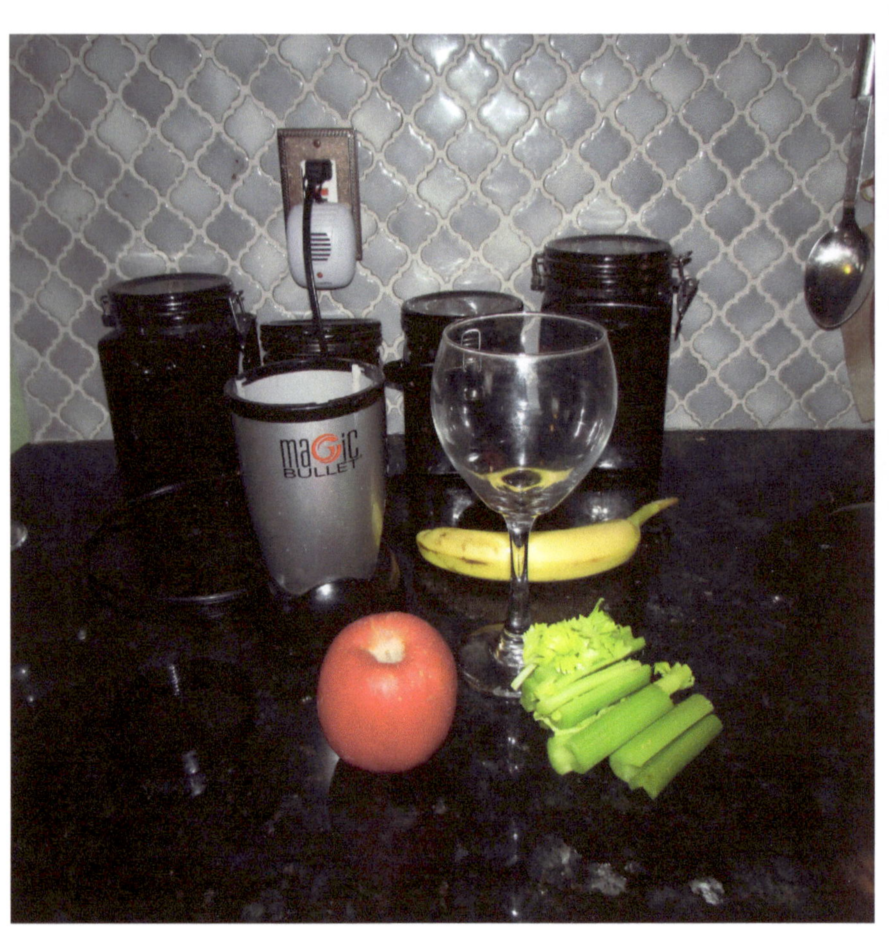

maGic
BULLET

If I am short of ingredients I use what I have. I still revert to the bullet blender a lot because I love the cups. I try to make 4 so I have enough for the day. I bought 4 extra and solid lids to go with them. My daughter has 5 lol. I like the bullet blender containers with handles. They don't spill as often and the handles help.

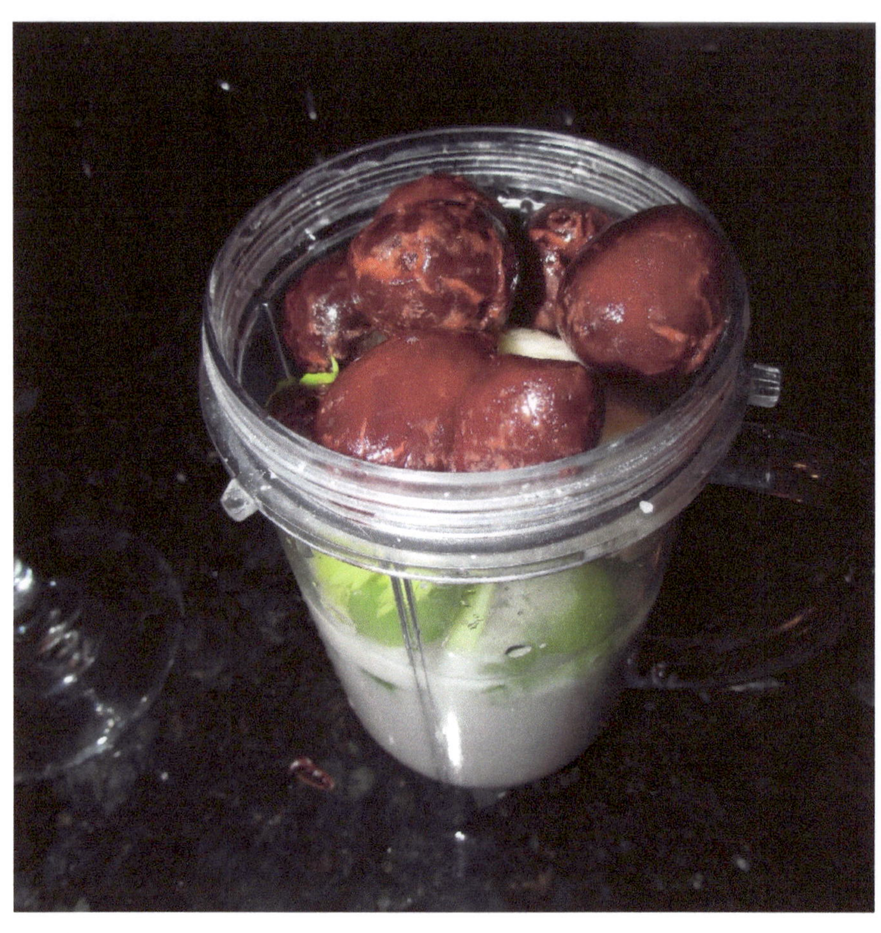

These are frozen cherries, celery, banana and cashew milk. The kids say it tastes like ice cream. I do freeze the bananas and cherries.

I don't measure anything. Some days I make it more liquid. I still use a bullet blender but we also use a Vitamix or Ninja Blender to make 4-5 smoothies at a time. They are both available on Amazon. I now use the large blender and put four bullet blender cups in the frig with smoothie for the next day.

I give them to other family members. My daughter takes 4 to work each day.

My daughter usually doesn't have time for lunch and this works great for her. My husband has begun to lose some weight. This is difficult for him because he eats a lot of sweets and meat. It is a struggle to change things for him. He is doing one meal replacement a day.

I have started the grandchildren on this. I give them a modified recipe and they are happy with that.

Their recipe is :

Children's Smoothie

Frozen bananas(I peel and cut and put in freezer)
Cashew Almond or Coconut milk
Celery or kale
frozen fruit

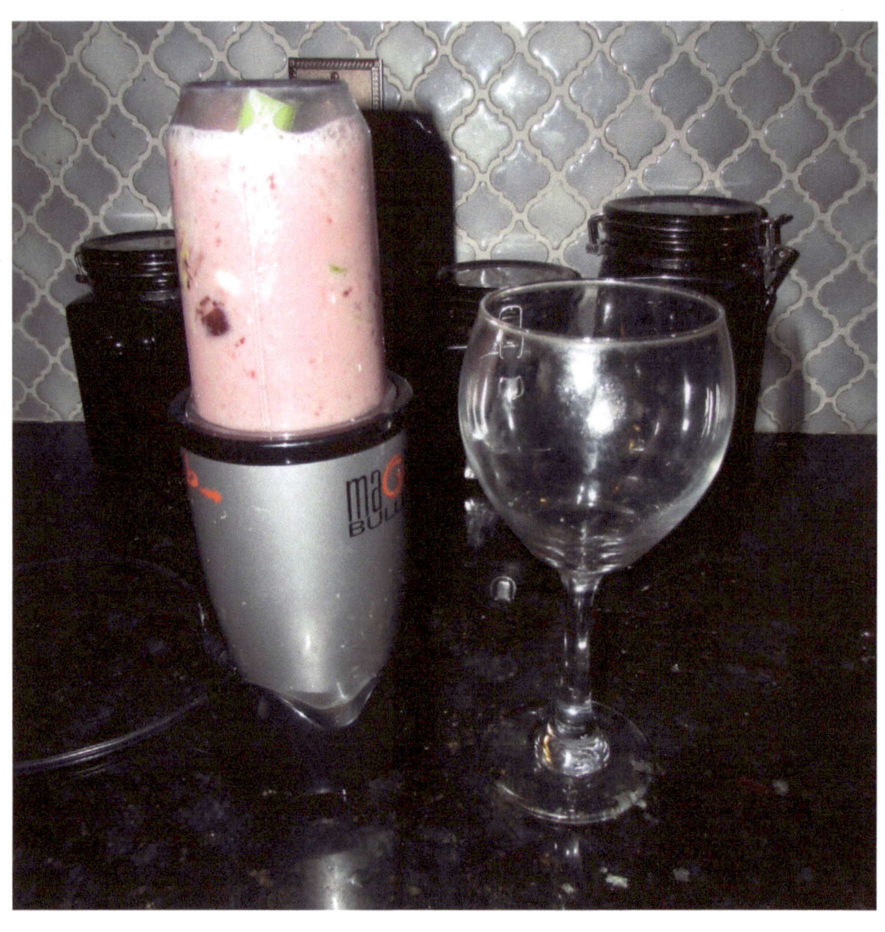

They normally love this and ask for more. They seem to get colds less often.

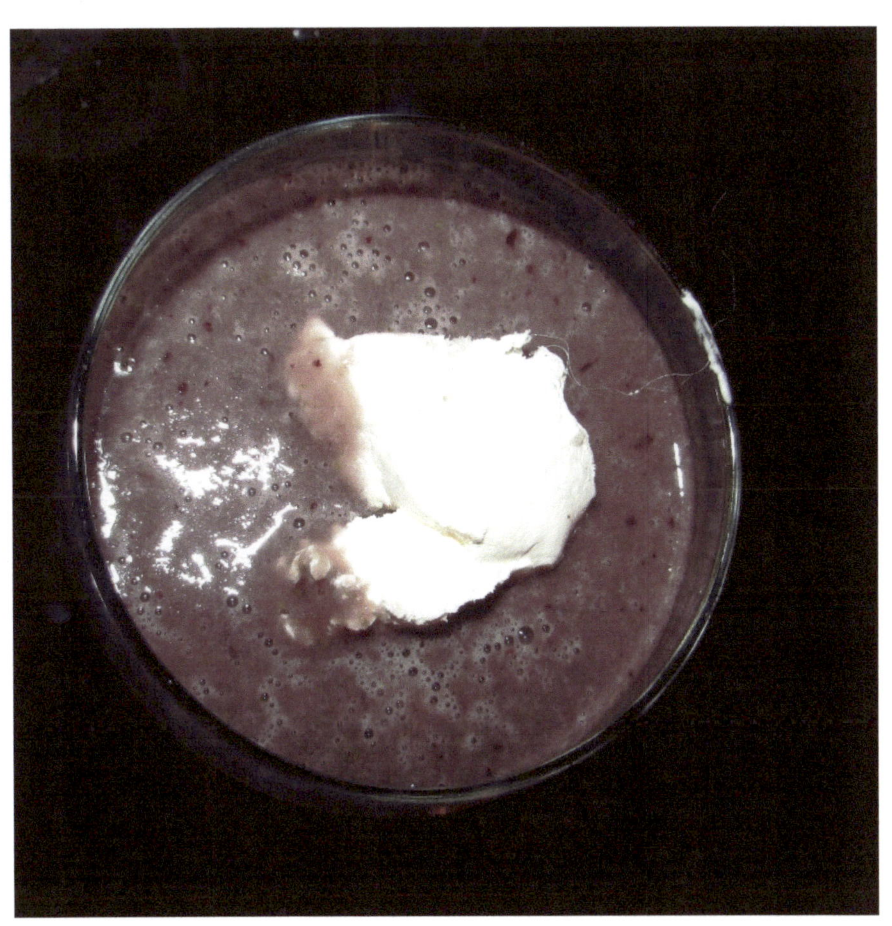

I added a bit of whipped cream to this. My mom lived to be over 90 and often did this. Look at the whipped cream. A small amount has very low calories and carbs. Low carbs are important. I use stevia but very little.

You can change the recipes for allergies or taste but make them vegan,low carb, and low calorie.

I have been only doing smoothies for breakfast.

I didn't lose much the first month but I felt healthier.

After about 6 weeks I weighed myself and I was surprised. I had lost 15 pounds. That really never happened to me before without starvation mode and I usually gained it back.

I was away for a while and hadn't weighed myself for a while again. When I did I had lost another 15 lbs. So altogether that's 30. I hadn't gained weight over the holidays. I now have lost another 5.

My goal is another 10 and to get more firm. I do an exercise glider and bike about 5 minutes a day . I was swimming and going to the gym. I was doing pilates. I know I should go back. I'm hoping to firm up a little. I had an ankle injury so that was hard but I try to fight it.

In short-I'm so surprised that I lost all this weight. I really like it too. I'm used to it now and it's easy. Another strange effect is my fingernails grow fast and are fantastic. In my whole life I have never had nails like this.

So I'm hoping to help others and I hope this works for you. Please share this.

I'm hoping I don't rebound. It has been 4 months plus minus so I'm hoping!!!!

I usually eat snacks like nuts and popcorn. Occasionally I eat a chocolate bar or ice cream. I eat one fairly big meal a day. I try to eat that for lunch. Here is my lunch today.

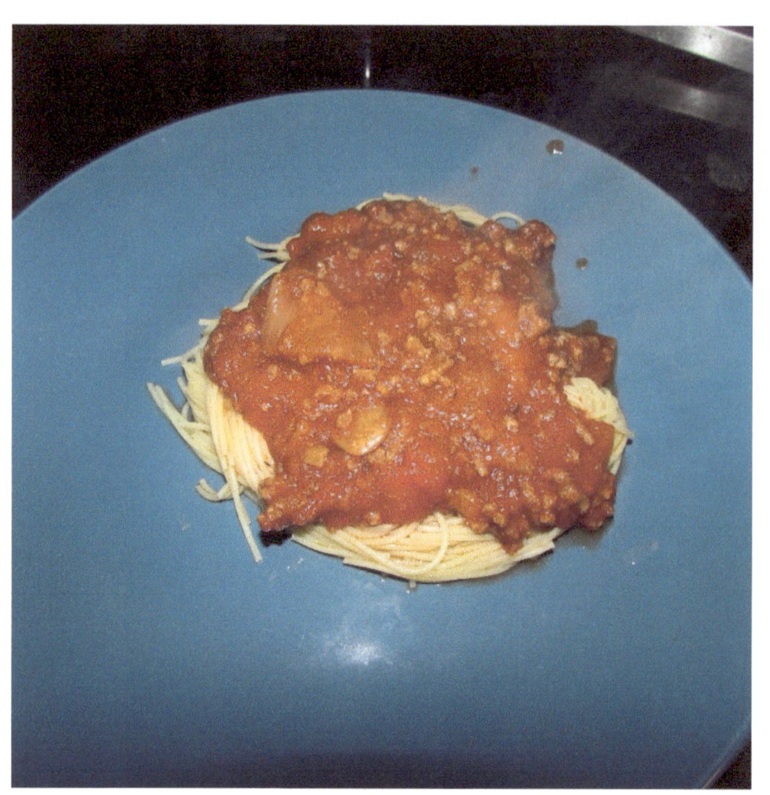

My lunch was pasta. Again I try to make it a smaller amount of meat or dairy. I caramelize 2 onions and 3 peppers diced. I cook 1 lb. low fat hamburger separately. I add pasta sauce and diced tomatoes to the carmelized peppers and onions. I then add all these together. This makes at least enough for 10 servings. Basically people are eating a tenth pound of meat but everyone loves it.

This is higher carb than I usually eat. If you want to really eat lower carbs eat only the sauce or a tiny tiny bit of pasta. I use high protein barilla pasta for less carbs, It's always gone and requested, so I guess the family likes it. You can just really cut down on the meat, dairy, and carbs.

The dairy is a bit difficult for me but there is vegan cheese and I love the cashew milk.

In short I've never
been able to lose weight
consistently and I am!!!!

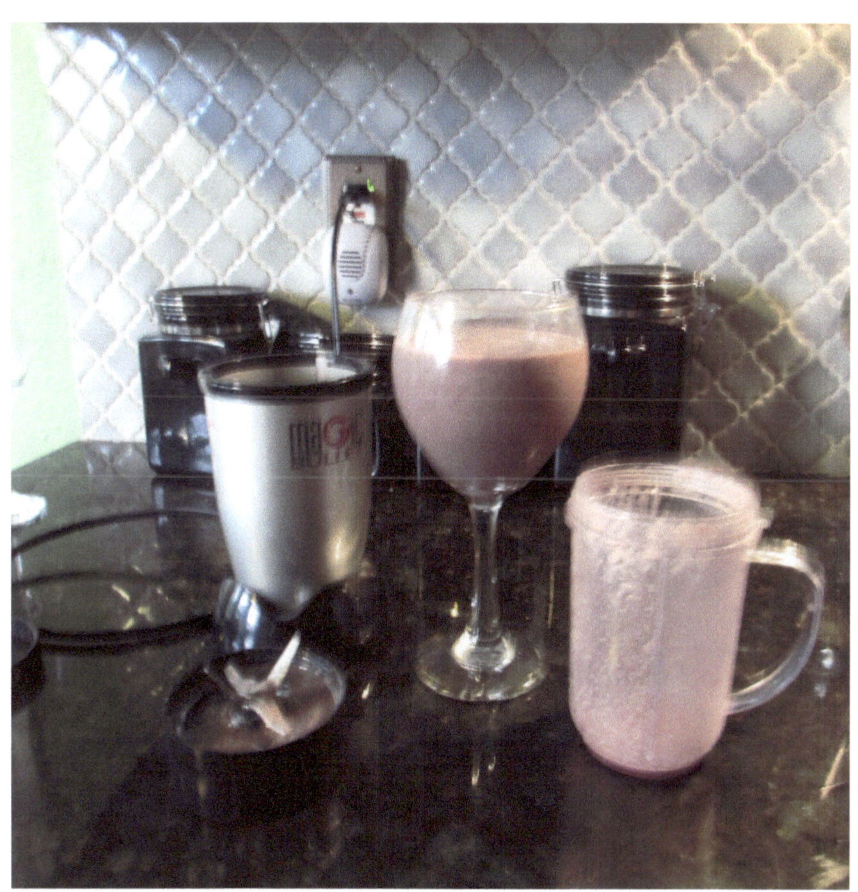

I'm going to 2 smoothies a day now. I really would like to be the weight I was at 25. Im within the top range of the BMI now so I'm finally in my BMI.

I'm wishing you the best of luck. If you cheat try to get back to it. Try to limit meat, dairy, and carbs. Try to eat lots of veggies and fish. I sometimes go off it for a few days if I don't have access to a blender. I still didn't gain weight.

Please feel free to e-mail me if I can help: sammygrammy2@gmail.com

Thanks for reading. I'll be adding more recipes to a new version. If you'd like to send me recipes and experiences please do.

I'm really hoping people can lower their sugar, weight, cholesterol, and help other health problems by eating more vegetables, less sugar, less alt, and less fat. Namaste and love to all.
Sammy Grammy

Please visit my site and click on amazon link to buy supplies.
https://sites.google.com/view/bookskeytoliteracy/home